The World of Slimming

One man's true life experience of going on a diet and
losing weight with Slimming World

Ken Jones

Acknowledgement: With grateful thanks to the members of Bluebrook Park Slimming World Group

Other books written by Ken Jones

Guilty Until Proven Innocent – *The tale of a man falsely accused*
The Memoirs of Edward Rochester – *'Jane Eyre' re-written by the man in the story*

Books by Naomi Davies

Sandy Wrighton and Friends – A series of short romantic novels

Healing Love
A Maldives Adventure
For The Love Of Music
The Welsh Victorian Dolls Mystery
The Absent Bridegroom

Colourblindness – The Unwritten Code – *A Parent's Guide to Colourblindness.*

ISBN-13: 978-1543186574
ISBN-10: 1543186572

Contact: TheWorldOfSlimming.com

Page set up and layout – KJPublishing.com

Contents

Foreword

I first met Ken and his lovely wife when my husband Daniel and I moved into Bracknell many years ago – a simple knock at their door at the time has led to a wonderful lifelong friendship that continues to this day. Ken is a great, down-to-earth individual with an incredible sense of humour and is full of mischief as you will see when you read through this book.

Having been through this weight loss journey myself (more for self-esteem rather than medical reasons in my case) I can confirm that Ken's story accurately reflects the experiences of many of our members on their weight loss journeys - the terror, the anticipation, the laughter, the tears and the absolute joy of getting to that *'Target'* weight.

As a Consultant reading this book, I have found Ken's perspective as a member of my group very enlightening. It has further reinforced how important my role is to encourage and support my members all the way to their dream weight-loss goals.

There is no doubt that if you are on a weight-loss journey with a group like ours you will be sharing the ups and downs that Ken experiences in this book. Know that no matter what may get in the way, whether you take the 'wiggly route' or the more 'direct route' to your personal Target, your determination, like Ken's, is what will get you through a very emotional and yes, mostly enjoyable journey. It will be full of friendship and love with a fantastic ending to look forward to.

I am sure that you will thoroughly enjoy this fascinating read.

Mandy-Lace

Introduction

This is the story of one man's foray into Slimming World. It is my diary record of what happened each week in my first year. It also reflects my feelings and opinions about the whole experience as I attended my group. Most of the incidents and events occurred just as they are written within these pages. I have, however, added and embellished details to make the flow of the book more entertaining and easier to read. There is also some fiction to a few of the anecdotes. They didn't always truly happen precisely as written but they could have done so, quite easily.

All the names have been changed to protect both the innocent and the guilty, although I am sure most regular members of the Bluebrook Park Slimming World group will be able to work out who everyone is. I have also altered some brand names and company names.

What started as a reluctant entrance into the world of slimming has resulted in an enthusiasm for eating well and living healthily. I am still quite unwell because of my major health scare in October 2015, but I am mercifully, still alive to tell the tale. This would not have been so had I not lost my weight and started exercising. I am particularly grateful to the following people.

Naomi – My wife of 38 years. I am very fortunate to have the wonderful Naomi with me.

Mandy-Lace – The Bluebrook Park Slimming World consultant. I will say much more about the excellent Mandy-Lace within the text of the book.

Dr Cody – My GP who helped me get started by funding my Slimming World subscription for 24 weeks. He is accessible, involved, and on my side. He also calls me from time to time on my mobile phone which is a surreal pleasure for me.

The Beloved Tamara – This is not one person. It is a blend of some of the nurses who cajoled and encouraged me to change my ways after my heart operation. They were not quite as brusque as I have portrayed although some days it came very close. The staff of Frimley Park Hospital rehabilitation program are magnificent.

The Bluebrook Park Slimming World Group members – Thank you for receiving me into your world and supporting me week by week.

Before proceeding with my diary, I should mention that I am a professional dieter of Olympic pedigree. I have been training for 35 years and successfully added eight and a half stones of extra weight to my masculine frame in that time. I hardly noticed what was going on. I defy you to name a diet that I have not tried. Low fat, high carb, ketonic, high fibre, meal replacement potions, 5-2 diet, 3-4 diet, hip and thigh diet, cabbage soup diet, et al.

Did the Slimming World diet work any better for me? Well it simply had to as I had no choice in the matter. It was diet or die! I did have hope that eating proper food and getting support from the group would make a difference.

Read on to discover what happened.

Week Minus Three – Doomed!

The hospital rehabilitation nurses had told me I needed to lose weight. They weren't even polite and nice about it. With a broad grin that disguised a major threat, I was told in no uncertain terms to change my ways or expect to die in the near future. The nurse in question, the beloved Tamara, seemed to take great pleasure in her work but I am not sure this pleasure was always best placed.

Over the twelve sessions of rehabilitation I witnessed the beloved Tamara bark out the same warning to most of the other patients as they joined and left the group. The rehab sessions were a mix of educational talks, thirty minutes of circuit training and then a cool down. The educational talks were just that, educational. Where else would you watch a series of brilliant presentations on looking after your heart after major surgery? The circuit training was light and easy in the first session, but quickly increased in difficulty over the weeks. Each session ended with what I called the 'spooky warm down'.

This was when the lights would be switched off and we were all told to sit in a circle with our eyes closed and follow the beloved Tamara's softly spoken instructions. They played weird ethereal music in this part of the session. I found myself sitting in a darkened room, full of strangers who had all had a major heart attack or incident in the previous few months. I was so relieved that we didn't have to hold hands and chant 'Is there anyone there?'.

"So how are you going to lose weight?" The beloved Tamara's diet inquisition began. Her own, shall we say without recrimination, 'Stocky' build, fought against the wisdom that proliferated from her own mouth. To be straightforward, it was a bit rich her telling me to lose weight when she had completely failed in this pursuit herself.

I magnanimously said nothing about this, hoping to preserve my life by patiently waiting for her to continue.

"There's no point you sitting there promising me you will improve your ways. I need to write down on our records what specific action you intend to take." Her eyes bulged out as if there was a hydraulic pump pushing air into her big eyes from the back of her head. I returned her expression with my own doleful look.

"What do you suggest?" As I asked, her breathlessness increased, evidenced by the cheeks joining her eyes with the pumpy puffing out thing.

"I expect people like you in my care *(Care? I think inwardly)* who have nearly died from a heart episode *(It was more than an episode to me!)* to take control and make your own decisions."

"But I am simply asking for an idea about what is a good diet." I thought she was going to completely explode because of the throbbing pump in her head.

At that very moment another patient, Trudi, decided to have a heart spasm and this distracted the beloved Tamara from further vilification of me and my ignorance. I was most grateful to Trudi for the interruption whilst hoping that she would quickly recover from her spasm and be well again. Trudi decided she wanted to go home and we never saw her at the rehab group again. She died a few days later.

At the end of the exercise session the beloved Tamara came over.

"We recommend you join Slimming World or Watchers of Weight."

"And do you have their numbers?"

"No! You are an adult. Look it up on Google."

Nice!

My nearest and dearest also showed the same rather extreme enthusiasm for me to lose weight. I recalled to her the instructions that I had been given by the nurses.

Give her full credit, without cheering out loud verbally or dancing down the garden path naked, I could tell that she agreed wholeheartedly with the advice given to me by the hospital.

Naomi even offered to come with me. Now my nearest and dearest could never in a million years be called overweight. *(Other than by the Slimming World consultant, Mandy-Lace, more of that later)*. I certainly wouldn't dare say such a thing.

But my nearest and dearest had expressed a desire to lose a small amount of weight. She also said that she wanted to support me in my struggle to lose weight. *'Drag me there by the goolies, more like!'* I mused inwardly. I still had some doubt about the honesty and integrity of my nearest and dearest's motives for accompanying me. Sometimes I thought she just wanted to make sure I attended the weekly sessions, and didn't run off to play snooker with my mates instead.

It fell to me to make the phone call. I left a respectable amount of time, ten days specifically, between receiving the *'Orders from on high'* and the multiple reminders from my nearest and dearest before looking up the number on Google. Then I saved the number on my mobile and waited for a further three days. I didn't want to appear too eager and rush into things. Something surprised me about the fact that the consultant's name given on the Slimming World website was Mandy-Lace. I remembered fondly a Mandy-Lace from the past as a beautiful and vivacious individual with a huge personality that always brought a cheer into a room. Surely it couldn't be the same person. I consulted with my nearest and dearest.

"The consultant's name is Mandy-Lace Weldon. There can't be many people in Bracknell with that name." My wife looked at me with hope. We had often wondered what had happened to our old friends Mandy-Lace and her husband Daniel. We hadn't seen them for years.

"I want it to be her." Naomi said with some hope. I echoed the feeling.

It was in fact the very same person. Just hearing her voice on the phone cheered me up no end. But at the same time, I tried to think of a way not to join the diet group without upsetting her. After all, I wasn't ever serious about following the advice of the beloved Tamara or my nearest and dearest.

"You must come!"

"Must I?"

"You will love it!"

"Will I?"

"Everyone is so friendly!"

"Are they?"

"I would love to see you and Naomi again, it's been so long since we had an evening together." This was a very underhand tactic to finally persuade me, but it worked. How could I turn down the beautiful Mandy-Lace? Impossible!

"How is Daniel?"

"Oh, he would love to see you again. We must get together as a foursome." Of course we must.

Then Mandy-Lace asked the fateful question.

"How did you find out about Slimming World?" I related to Mandy-Lace the experiences of the previous four months ending with me lying on an operating theatre table having heart surgery. This was the first time I had vocalised my experiences out loud to another person. My nearest and dearest had witnessed the saga first hand but now I was telling my own story. It was a curiously moving experience. It felt as if I was talking about someone else, but as I reached the end of my sorry tale I knew the truth of it in my own mind. I needed help and speaking about my illness out loud for the very first time cemented this knowledge into my thick skull.

"Where do you hold the meetings?"

"We hold them in Bluebrook Park Hall every Saturday morning. Do you know it?"

"My house backs onto Bluebrook Park." The sense of inevitability was oppressive and stifling. I took a deep breath.

"What time on Saturday?"

"Nine o'clock in the morning for about an hour and a half." Hmm. I wouldn't even lose an evening in the week and still have nearly the whole weekend free.

"Because of what you have told me I think that there is a possibility that your doctor might pay your fees for the first three months."

"Really? Why would he do that?"

"A lot of people are referred to our group by their doctor. It is quite a regular thing."

"I already have a check-up booked on Monday. I'll ask Dr Cody." I was sure that he wouldn't pay for me...

Monday's Doctor Appointment

..."Of course, we will give you a referral and pay for you, and if you are successful in losing weight then I will give you a second voucher for another three months. But six months is the maximum."

Result!

"Oh no, six months is great, thanks." My mind was full of doubts as I headed headlong and unavoidably towards the Slimming World diet for myself.

I considered my situation. I knew the consultant personally; the meeting was held a few yards from my front door and my doctor was prepared to pay for me for up to six months. There was no escape. I was doomed to enter Slimming World!

Week Minus Two – Nearest and Dearest

"How was it?" Naomi had decided to start her Slimming World experience before me, such was her eagerness and determination to ensure my future participation. I was still waiting for my referral voucher to come in the post. As a reconnaissance mission, I thought that it would be useful and informative for us both if she checked out Slimming World in preparation for my joining. A small part of me hoped that my nearest and dearest had endured an hour and a half of hell and would try and talk me out of joining Slimming World.

"Fantastic! You will love it!" She was alive and glowing as she told me all about the people in the group and how everything happened. It sounded dreadful as I heard about being weighed and clapped and talking about how you were doing with the diet. There was a definite *'But'* in her voice that I spotted early on in the conversation. She finished telling me about how fantastic it all was, and then a darkness spread over her face. I stayed silent and asked the question with a simple, silent sideways move of my head and a raise of my eyebrows.

"I've just got weighed, you won't believe how heavy I am." I regarded my wife's body seriously and wondered if it were true. She had never been very big but we both knew that she had put on a few pounds over the years. I could see the disappointment in her eyes.

"OK, so we are both going to do this." She nodded back quietly, blinking her tears away.

She had been given an A5 double plastic folder full of information booklets about Slimming World. I eagerly devoured them over a decidedly non-slimming lunch of Takeaway Pizza and garlic bread with wedges and chilli dip.

I have still not received the voucher in the post for me to join up.

Week Minus One – Waiting Patiently!

No voucher!

No group!

No diet!

No weight loss!

Nothing!

Grrrr!

Week Zero – Abject Terror

It was never going to be the happiest entrance I had ever made. How bad could it be? Well as it turned out, it was dreadful! My nearest and dearest having already attended for the last two weeks had offered me comfort and encouragement of a sort. But now I was being dragged along to the group. It takes 127 seconds for me to walk begrudgingly from my front door to the door of Bluebrook Park Hall. I timed it, twice! It takes 59 seconds to walk home by the same route.

There were signs outside the hall with arrows pointing towards the entrance saying *'Fat People This Way!'*. OK they didn't say that, but it felt like it. Then on reaching the inner door to the hall there was a stand-up promotional sign with cut out people scowling and looking miserable at having to join Slimming World. OK, they looked disgustingly happy and cheerful. I'm just saying how I felt.

I hoped that no one would notice me or make a fuss as I reluctantly and nervously entered the room, but that didn't work out at all. Mandy-Lace was primed and well prepared by my nearest and dearest. She was ready with a loud exclamation of joy and a huge, enthusiastic hug.

"This is the lovely Ken who I have known for many years." She announced to the onlooking crowd of big people. She grabbed me by the hand and led me to a curved line of chairs which was apparently the *'New Members'* area. Mandy-Lace gloriously and efficiently talked me through the ins and outs of how to succeed with the Slimming World eating system. I was quite bright and clever at school many years ago, being good at quadratic equations and calculus, but this day I couldn't understand a word of what she was saying. My mind was on other things.

There were indeed, many distractions within the Bluebrook Park Hall. People were queuing up in one part of the room to pay their sub fees and other people were getting weighed.

Some were giving each other high fives and cheering having lost weight, Others were mournfully and quietly getting off the scales having found out that they had put weight on. I could feel their pain from a distance of 6 metres away. Everyone was cheerful and welcoming apart from those who had not lost weight. Those members looked like they were about to attend their own funeral. One of them glanced across towards me with murderous intent.

Then came the talk session and the clapping. Every achievement was applauded and almost cheered by the whole of the group. I quickly decided that in order to preserve my fingers for my guitar playing I would only clap a little for each person. Nevertheless, it became apparent that some of the big people in the room used to be a whole lot bigger. They were reporting huge weight losses as Mandy-Lace worked around the room. No one escaped their turn apart from me as it was my first week. I had not yet been weighed.

I'm now going to share about the weighing machine. I spotted it very early on in my short time in the municipal hall. The machine was heavy duty and black in colour. It stood on four feet, one on each corner. It looked at me across the room threateningly. At one point, I'm sure I saw the machine stand up on these feet and come towards me saying *'I'm coming to get you!'*. Then I looked again and thought that it was looking at me with an evil smile and the wink of an eye. Weighing machines have many eyes, they know what you have been eating and how much exercise you have been doing. At the end of the meeting I knew that there was no turning back. I handed my doctor's voucher over and approached the bench. The verdict was going to be guilty, but how harsh was the sentence going to be?

In the introduction of her talk, Mandy-Lace said to the group "We don't do blame or shame here." Well today for me, reading the scales, and knowing that the ladies monitoring the scales knew the true horror of my full weight, I felt both shameful and blameful.

I was responsible for my brush with life and death and now I knew the scale of the task ahead of me.

Terrifying!

Footnote: There are some weeks when nearly every one fails to lose weight. These are the weeks when the weighing machine is broken. Mandy-Lace never believes the members about this malfunction and insists that the scales have been accurately calibrated. But we as members know better than that. Some weeks the machine is broken. That is my opinion and I am sticking to it.

Week One - This Was Never Going To Work

"I'm not doing anything different to what we do normally, so how on earth am I going to lose weight on this stupid diet?" I was looking for my nearest and dearest to confirm my opinion. No such luck!

"Well we haven't had takeaway this week and we are not doing much frying of food. And you have hardly eaten any bread this week. We have reduced our wine intake to one glass a day so that should help us both." We had both dramatically reduced our alcohol intake as there was a nasty leaflet in the new members' pack about not drinking too much. The beloved Tamara at the hospital never mentioned the lack of alcohol. The big difference with our food was the amount of fruit and vegetables we were enduring/enjoying with all our meals.

I had learnt on my first group meeting that most vegetables and fruit were called 'speed foods'. I mistakenly thought this meant that by simply adding them to our meals they would somehow and rather magically neutralise the weight loading effects of the rest of the food on my plate. It took many weeks for me to discover and correct this major error.

But there was more confusion for me with the Healthy 'A's and Healthy 'B's. It sounded to me as confusing as a British Rail train timetable. You can have one Healthy 'A' a day but if you have already had it you can 'Syn' any more that you have. You can also have one Healthy 'B' per day. But you have to 'Syn' any other ones you eat.

I looked up in my book to see if things were different on a Tuesday but there was nothing about this in any of the books. Further to this there was something called Extra Easy Speed week where you could have two Healthy 'B's per day, I still have no idea what all this means. I'll try and work it out and explain in a later diary entry. (See Week Thirty-Nine).

Week Two – Unbelievable!

I wasn't expecting that. Six and a half pounds lost in the first week. I love Slimming World! It's my favourite thing in the whole world! At this rate, I will be done with the dieting in a few weeks. Some members rejoiced with me at the weight loss. Others looked on sagely with a knowing smile. I know this look now but it was new to me back then. I have been practicing my own version of 'the look' in the mirror for when I get to be a Slimming World 'know it all'. Not there yet.

I noticed a strange phenomenon this week. Some people get weighed and leave the group immediately. This is a puzzle to me. I decide to observe this from week to week and see what is happening. I can't understand why you would pay to come to group to get help and then go home without getting what you paid for. A mystery to ponder.

The forensic examination of everybody's successes and failures was much more interesting this week as I had my own amazing loss to brag about. When Mandy-Lace came to talk about me she was gushing and overwhelming in her praise for me. I could feel my face redden up and I wished I could disappear. I usually like being the centre of attention but on this occasion, I hardly knew what to say or do. Apparently, I am *'Fabulous!'*

Everything about the Slimming World experience still feels very new and fresh. I spotted today that some people are wearing Slimming World branded T shirts and polo shirts. Very swish. These people are assisting with the pay station and where people get weighed. They are very involved in everything that goes on.

Something about the great atmosphere in the room gives me confidence that I will succeed with this diet. Mandy-Lace made it very clear to me that the diet does work if you follow the food optimizing eating plan.

Week Three – Still Not Getting It

The voyage of discovery continues. I think I understand the diet and then I discover that I have got it wrong completely. I am totally missing homemade freshly baked cakes enormously. I moaned about this in the group to a quiet murmur of sorrowful agreement.

There doesn't seem to be many really good cake recipes in any of the information packs. No one mentions chocolate cake or doughnuts when they discuss their food choices.

I have tried out some of the Slimming World main course recipes from a book that I won last week. I can't recall how I won the book. The recipes are all nice and tasty but need spicing up a bit. That is not a problem as apparently, I can treat herbs and spices as free foods.

I keep forgetting to fill in the food diary that I must submit each week. I have also decided not to write everything down as it is a secret and I do not want Mandy-Lace to know about it. I had a beer after playing snooker on Wednesday which was free as I didn't record it. I also pinched a slice of pizza that my son cruelly waved beneath my nose late one evening. He is busy trying to put weight on. It is an easy life for some. The slice of pizza was quite delicious and also free.

The other element to the Slimming World diet is exercise. They call it *'Body Magic'*. I think that I would be good at this part of the plan but my heart will not let me participate fully as yet. I plan to increase my exercise as soon as I can. There are some members who are doing lots of exercise. Running 10k runs and going to the gym. I am only allowed to walk. I have started walking around Bracknell but my limit is about two miles. After that I am pooped.

Week Four – She Suspects

Mandy-Lace quizzed me searchingly and persistently about the food diary I submitted last week. She suspects me of cheating! I decided to lie and told her I was a complete paragon of virtue with the food diaries. Next week's one will be the last I must complete. Then they are optional.

I had a heart to heart with June, one of the other members of the group. I explained that I had cheated with the food diary. It turns out that she is a co-conspirator in this. She doesn't record any chocolate that she eats. Quite brilliant! June further explained that any extras we eat should be called "Syns" and recorded on the form. I had wondered what the last column on the form was for. (I now know that 'Syns' stands for Synergy. It's a way of enjoying foods that many diets don't allow. See Week Thirty-Nine).

I like June. She thinks like me regarding being dishonest about the food we eat. But I prefer the spelling 'Sins'. I understand that word better and it reflects more accurately how I feel when I have extra food without writing it down.

Over the weeks, I have become quite friendly with some of the members and there is a good feeling of being together in our weight loss trial. But there are very few men in the group. The ones that are there seem nice and slim. I am the big one.

Mercifully a new chap, Phillip, joined today who is even larger than me. Hooray! I welcomed him warmly and introduced him to Mandy-Lace. 'He won't last' I thought to myself. How wrong I was. Why am I so negative about other people's attitudes and reasons for wanting to lose weight? And why do I condemn them when I am just the same? I confess I am still working on this even now, but I am improving.

Week Five – Yes!

One Stone Award!

That is one stone of weight lost and gone forever.

Yes!
Yes!
Yes!
Yes!
Yes!

And a thousand times Yes!!!

Week Six – Utter Failure

Following the glory and the pride of last week's weight loss I came across a new word to describe myself this week. Maintained! The girl who was writing in my record book, Cherie, looked up with a warm smile as I stepped off the scales. I felt like I would continue going downwards and be swallowed down into the floor. It's all right for Cherie, she has almost finished losing weight and is nearly at her target weight. I'm beginning to feel the size of the huge task ahead of me.

Maintained! It seems such an innocent word when looked at on its own but it is full of unpleasant meaning. It also expresses what I haven't done. I haven't maintained my eating program. I haven't maintained my concentration. I haven't maintained my good intentions. I knew this before I mounted the scales, but ridiculously thought that I could magically get away with it.

I moodily sat through the meeting which I now know is called *'Image Therapy'*. Mandy-Lace has a tablet computer which seems to hold all manner of secret information about me. She knows how much I have lost in weight and how much for just this week. She also knows when it is someone's birthday. The image of me sitting and sulking in the chair must have been obvious, as Mandy-Lace was very brief in her talk to me. I resolved to escape quickly at the end so that I could avoid being spoken to, one to one.

"Ken? Have you got a minute?"

'I've got all day but I still don't want to be spoken to.' I thought to myself. My nearest and dearest was laughing and chatting easily across the other side of the room and obviously was not ready to go home just yet. I sat down in my naughty seat and awaited the expected reprimand. It didn't come.

"Do not worry. A maintain happens to all of us every now and then. Just stick to what you are doing and you will be fine."

"Oh. Okay. Thanks Mandy-Lace."

"No problem" She gave me a friendly hug and went to see another member who was waiting to talk to her. I like Mandy-Lace.

'So now I feel guilty because she is so nice to me, even though I know in my heart of hearts that I could have followed the diet better in the last week.' I took my nearest and dearest out for dinner to recover my mood. Dinner out is great for some things but rotten for helping me lose weight. Ho Hum. Tomorrow is another day.

Week Seven – Special People

I am now part of the group. I know many of the regulars by name and share jokes and life with them easily. There are a few stand out people that have impressed themselves on my heart and mind in these early weeks.

Naomi – My nearest and dearest who tries to be subtle with her encouragement from day to day and fails every time. She is desperate for me to lose my weight and live a full and long life. She wants it more than I do.

Mandy-Lace – My Slimming World consultant. Why did we ever stop being friends? How did we drift apart? We are now friends for life.

Samantha – Was awarded her three stone award this week. I am totally in awe of her success.

Tom and Bindi – This married couple have both reached their weight loss target and yet still come to the group to keep them on the straight and narrow. Tom sells raffle tickets that fund the free coffee and tea we have in group. More of this another time. Bindi attends the stripping section and makes sure there is a good flow of bodies in line ready to be weighed. More of this another time also. Tom and Bindi are very important members of the group for lots of reasons.

Phillip – Already an integral part of the group even though he joined a mere three weeks ago. We sit together at the back and make sideways comments throughout the '*Image Therapy*' hour. His early weight loss is better than mine which is infuriating but I can't dislike him for that. I sense competition.

Zena – Zena is the daughter of a man I knew forty-five years ago, as a teenager. Her character, conversation and quiet humour is just the same as his was all those years ago, and it is both unnerving and amusing for me to hear it coming out of her mouth.

We immediately hit it off and frequently hold up proceedings because we won't stop chatting. Her mum, Gillian, also comes and it is pleasing to know that my old friend found a good helpmate for himself.

Bert – Bert doesn't stay to the meetings but just comes to get weighed. I can't quite understand this and subsequently spend the whole year trying to get him to stay. We immediately have a bond when I discover that he lost his best friend to an unexpected and untimely illness two years previously. I tell him that I also had lost my best mate to pancreatic cancer and we understand everything about each other's pain without further discussion. Nothing more to say.

June – As previously mentioned I feel like we are conspirators on the same journey (Note: it took me till now to use the 'J' word). We also hold up the queue with our conversation. Quietly and very unassumingly June is losing a lot of weight week by week. I decided to align myself with her as she obviously knows how to do the Slimming World diet better than me.

There are many more special people but these are the people who became my inspiration and good friends over my first year. Much of my success is down to the support, friendship and encouragement of these special people.

Week Eight – Walking Magic

The hospital rehab nurses told me that the only exercise I am allowed to do is walking. No cycling or swimming and definitely no competitive sports. And boy have I been walking. I started with a few miles every now and then. I have now got up to 4 miles a day as a minimum. Mandy-Lace says that I will win more awards if I keep walking. I do not know why this matters to me because the awards are just stickers and bits of card and paper but I want to win awards. My resolve is further strengthened by the promise of the body magic awards. Over the following weeks, I race through Bronze, Silver and Gold Awards and eventually achieve a Platinum Award which means that exercise is an integral part of my life – which it now is.

I have a walking buddy, Rafe, who I walk with every Tuesday evening. We hardly knew each other when we started our walks, but we quickly became good friends over the year.

After about five months of walking, (Week Nineteen in this diary) I decided to email my GP to see if I was allowed to swim and cycle, now I had started losing weight.

He called me on my mobile phone the following morning.

"Hello Mr Jones, Ken?" He is always nervous to use my first name even though I said he could before.

"Yes?"

"This is Dr Cody. I got your email and wanted to talk to you about it. How are things going?"

"I have lost nearly three stones and am walking most days."

"You sound out of breath, are you alright?"

"I'm fine. I'm walking to Bracknell from Bagshot through Swinley Forest."

"But that must be seven miles or so."

"Yes it is."

"And you feel you can cope with that do you?"

"Yes I do."

"Well I'm sure you can start swimming and cycling now. You are doing much better than I anticipated. Just start slowly and build up your stamina."

"Thank you. And thank you for paying for me to do the Slimming World diet."

"In your case it is obviously money well spent."

"Yes it is."

"Well I'll leave you to your walk. Goodbye".

"Goodbye". I looked at the screen of my mobile phone in amazement. My own GP had called me personally on my mobile to tell me the good news. A most surreal, surprising and pleasing event.

We eagerly went swimming on Friday to discover that I could barely manage six lengths of the pool. I had to rest after every length. This was very disappointing as I used to swim for miles.

Week Nine – The Stripper

When you join up to Slimming World you quickly learn that what you wear to group is important. It affects the scales reading. If you wear heavy clothes you weigh more. It took me nine weeks to work this out. Week by week I would throw anything on in the rush to get out of the house and go to group not giving a thought to this aspect of the weigh in. I am much wiser now.

To help me work out my lightest outfit I carefully weighed my shirts and trousers this morning on the kitchen scales before group to ensure that my clothes were as light as possible. It worked. I'm sure it worked. It did work, didn't it?

I am not going to discuss the week I went *'commando'*. Never to be repeated. Stupid idea!

But there is a problem with the clothes and weighing in. Everyone takes off as much as possible to be as light as possible for the weigh in. I was initially shocked to see all the members easily stripping off their outer garments to get weighed and then getting re-dressed. However, there was always a sense of decency and decorum about it. No one stares and in fact everyone is still properly dressed to be weighed. After a few weeks, you hardly notice it is happening.

This was until one week when we had a visiting person to our group. She couldn't attend her own group that week so had decided to grace us with her presence. She proceeded to strip down to what could best be described as a body stocking. Sure enough, everything was covered, just, but it was hard not to stare. I was not staring in admiration, more a feeling of shock and dismay. There was a lot of body squeezed into her tight, semi-sheer outfit.

My distress made me unable to discuss the incident with anyone until now.

Week Ten – I Give Up

A black day. I can hardly articulate the punishing disappointment of putting weight on. So I won't. Dark, dark, dark days.

All is dark.

Naaaaaaaarrrrhhhhhhhhhhhh!!!!!!!!!!!!!!!!!

Week Eleven – Martina and Clarice

I now have the job of *Welcomer*. I wear one of those nice Slimming World branded polo shirts I mentioned earlier. I stand by the door and my role is to welcome people as they arrive. I must also try to spot newcomers to the group. This is part of my responsibility as a member of the social team. I try to work out who is a new person. These new people are taken by me to the new members' area to meet Mandy-Lace. Simple! Well not as simple as you would think.

There are so many regular members that I can't remember them all, let alone spot whether they are new to our group. And they all wear different outfits every week, just to confuse me more. Some new people walk straight in saying 'I'm new'. But most new people walk towards the door with fear and uncertainty. I can usually spot the worried look on their faces now, but I still miss a few which is maddening for me and hard on them.

Today two young ladies appeared who were new to our group but not new to Slimming World. I didn't know where to take them. Fortunately, they seemed to know the score and what to do. I have to say that mingling and talking with young ladies is not something I do very often but these two were just plain lovely people and very easy going. They knew where to go and I left them to it.

It turned out that Martina and Clarice were transferring to our group from another group and had been doing Slimming World for a couple of years. It also transpired that they had both lost a lot of weight in the past. When Mandy-Lace told us their weight losses during the *'Image Therapy'* session there was a communal intake of breath in amazement. There was something different and very attractive about these two young girls. They were positive and cheerful and had no edge or bad attitude about them.

I know that many existing members were drawn to them straightaway, as I was. Over the months since they joined the Bluebrook Park group they have been a positive influence for good in the group. Very inspiring.

It reminded me that how I behave and act towards other people has a major influence on them, and also on me. Attitude matters.

Week Twelve – We Are Talking Two Stones!

Very pleased. Two stones is a lot more than one. In fact, it is double the loss. Stones in plural, gone!

I can't remove the stupid, inane grin from my face. I bore people silly with the news as they queue up to pay their subs. Phillip and June are very generous with their kind words. Mandy-Lace makes a big fuss of me. Being an old hand at this now I do not blush or get bashful, but I realise how disappointed I would have been if my milestone had not been properly acknowledged. I am a child at heart as I receive my Two Stone Award with pleasure.

The only problem is that I have hardly started. I still have 5 stones to go to my 'Interim' target. I set this goal in the first week. I know that I will still need to lose another stone and a bit once I achieve my target. But one step at a time. If I were to lose seven stones that would be ridiculously amazing. For now, the first two stones feels very good indeed.

Today I noticed Candice and Laurie for the first time. They are another mother and daughter team who are determined to lose weight. This week a very frustrated Laurie let rip with her feelings about putting weight on having carefully followed the diet all week. The room was full of understanding. It was the first time I had heard someone really express their pain when things don't work out as we expect them.

I thanked Laurie for speaking out after the group meeting and told her that we all feel the same at times. I'm sure she didn't hear a word of what I said. I tried my best. It is bad weeks like this that show me how much I need the support of the other members in the group. Only two weeks ago, I felt exactly the same misery as Laurie. I wasn't forthright enough to speak my mind to the group as Laurie was. I hope she sticks with it. Her mum, Candice, for her part is pound by pound doing very well on the diet.

Week Thirteen – Shopping Is a Sensitive Subject

As I arrived at the supermarket to do my main food shop this week I passed a Slimming World member called Sophie coming out of the store as I was going in. She had a trolley fully laden with carrier bags and who knows what booty they contained? She almost screamed at the sight of me.

"Don't you look in my shopping bags!" Sophie moved swiftly to close the tops of the bags so that I could not see what contraband she was carrying. We both laughed at her predicament and I smiled as we passed each other knowing that I am also a bit touchy about being spotted shopping. It doesn't help that another member, Fern, works in the delicatessen section and is quite forthright and open about inspecting the contents of my shopping trolley. She will pass comment on anything that she disapproves of. I now avoid the delicatessen section entirely and buy cold meat from the pre-packed section.

The other embarrassing thing that happens is that when I casually meet another member doing their shopping it is impossible not to look judgmentally into their trolley. My first instinct is to look down and see what they are buying. It's like being a peeping Tom. Not that I have any experience of being one. *'What have you got in there that you shouldn't have?'* I ask without saying it out loud. Then I start making excuses for what I have bought hoping I haven't got to the wine department yet. It is so difficult and awkward that I find it best to shop at seven thirty in the morning when no one else is around.

When I do go at a busy time I always do a short reconnaissance of my chosen shopping aisle before entering it. I mumble the injunction *'Clear!'* to myself as I continue my shopping.

A similar problem occurs when you are eating out at a restaurant. You end up praying that no one will spot that you have ordered burger and chips even though you are on a diet.

Naomi, my nearest and dearest, is merciless when I order the wrong things.

"Mandy-Lace will find out about this."

"And how will that happen?"

"Because I will tell on you."

Snitch!

As we eat out so rarely I have no compunction about ordering what I want. The healthy options never taste as good. Whoever enjoys roast beetroot and squash salad in preference to burger and chips? Not me!

Week Fourteen – Cheating

"How do I love thee? Let me count the ways." – Sonnet 43 – Elizabeth Barratt Browning 1806 – 1861

There are many ways of cheating on the Slimming World diet. I love the simple elegance of these cheating methods. Some are plain and simply stupid. Others are more subtle, dubious and underhand. My experience is that if I cheat I stop losing weight. The anticipated spectre of the inevitable weekly weigh-in is a help to keeping me on the eating plan but sometimes I am an idiot and think that I can get away with a cheat. I have never got away with it. Ever! It always comes back to bite me on the scales.

All of these methods sabotage my weight loss. There are days when I feel compelled to cheat. I have little or no control over it. How do I love cheating? Let me count the ways. Here are my top seven cheating methods.

Cheating Method 1 – The Blast Furnace

This is where a rubbish event in your life gives you the mandate to forget that you were ever on a diet in the first place. Or at least, this is the way it makes you feel when you come up against real life situations. This could be the death of someone close, relationship problems, or simply a bad day at the office. You erase your memory files and common sense and decide to forget your diet completely. You even shop especially so that you can eat all the foods you have been missing. No one ever missed a piece of lettuce or a stick of celery. But alcohol, crisps, chocolate, peanuts, cakes, cookies, beef steak and giant burgers are what most people miss.

The important thing with the blast furnace cheating method is to completely go for it so that you are physically vomiting everything back up.

Then after a wash and brush up you can continue with your mega binge.

Professional dieters like me can successfully put on a good seven pounds in one day with a prolonged session of the Blast Furnace method.

Cheating Method 2 – The Exocet Missile

This is a method of cheating where you don't have to feel as guilty. It's not your fault. It's where you are innocently getting on with your life and your Slimming World plan when some gloriously unhealthy, fattening food presents itself. You didn't plan it and you weren't expecting it. This could be at a works leaving party or a social event.

It could even be in the sports centre café. This is a nice touch because you can justify your cheating by saying to your brain that you have earned the cheat because you have exercised. And after all this is in a sports centre. I still don't understand the fact that sports centres serve unhealthy foods. That's a discussion for another day.

The point is that the Exocet missile was unexpected and closely targeted towards you. Because of that you weren't ready to resist the temptation. You were caught unawares. If you want to escape the Exocet missiles you must be mentally prepared at all times for whatever could happen at any point of the day.

This takes a lot of practice. You must coach yourself to not partake of any food that you did not plan for. You must plan for every eventuality. If there is a chance on a Friday that someone is going to bring a birthday cake in, rehearse your lines and have your own lunch ready to hand. Easy to say, hard to do.

Cheating Method 3 – The Secret Eater

I do most of the food shopping for my nearest and dearest and myself. This can lead to secret purchasing of snacks and foods. The journey in the car from my local supermarket to home takes about seven minutes.

It is possible to eat 200g of salted peanuts and a 100g bar of milk chocolate in this time. I'm not telling you how I know this, but it has been properly researched more than once. What is more, you can hide the evidence of the wrappers in the green bin before you enter the house. No one will ever know. Other than Naomi who is like a forensic scientist when it comes to my cheating. She knows it all.

Now that I walk a lot more there is even more time to eat secretly when I walk to and from the local supermarket. But eating and walking at the same time gives me indigestion so I can't do this method of cheating successfully. Each to his own.

Cheating Method 4 – Falling off the Wagon

I find this the hardest cheating method to guard against. You are following the Slimming World diet and everything is hunky dory when something in your brain 'clicks' and you simply have to have a certain food item. This is a bit like cravings that pregnant women have (I think!). There is often no logic about what you actually crave. But you know in your mind that you must have some, whatever your poison is, before you return to your diet. You can't live another day without your favourite food.

Most times I simply submit to the craving and then move on. I do not have a strategy to stop this type of craving as yet. I'm working on it.

Cheating Method 5 – Double/Extra Portion

This one is brilliantly subtle. You know that you are eating good heathy food and decide to have a double portion. Or just a little bit more. The thinking goes like this. *'If I eat this Slimming World Chilli and Rice dinner again I will lose weight twice as fast.'* There is a fatal flaw in this. You have just doubled your calorie intake for that meal.

A more insidious version is where you simply add extras to every meal. Your porridge oats in the morning is 50 grams instead of 40 grams. Then your lunch time salad has four pieces of meat instead of two. Your evening dinner meal has some left overs that you do not want to waste so you eat it for supper.

Cheating Method 6 – Justified

Here is what happens. You are angelic all week, not swaying from your eating plan and then you get weighed. Horror of horrors, you have put weight on. It seems impossible that this could have happened. This sometimes occurs on a week when the machine is broken (See Week Zero) but normally it is just plain bad luck.

You say to yourself *'What's the point, I was good last week so I am going to ****** **** eat what I like this week. This stupid diet doesn't work anyway.'* You justify your cheating and create a self-fulfilling prophecy about your next week's weigh. When you come to the following week's group you say to Mandy-Lace 'I've had a bad week' and get on the scales. What would you know! You put on yet another few pounds.

Note: Sometimes you miraculously dodge a bullet and still lose weight even though you know you have eaten off plan. In my experience the cheating will eventually come back to bite you. You haven't escaped the consequences of your actions in the long term. It will get you in the end.

Cheating Method 7 – Flexible Syns

This is supposed to be the right way to party and still not overdo things. The idea is that you set your Syns for an event and stick to it. I did this for a summer barbeque in June with a target of 30 Syns. I had smashed this number by eight thirty in the evening and ended up hitting 98 Syns for the night out. Counting them was almost fun.

Mandy-Lace says that you can't carry the Syns over to the next day. It doesn't work like that. I wish it did.

The obvious problem with Flexible Syns for me is that it requires willpower. **I still do not have this elusive gift.** It would be better for me to refuse all food and drink for the evening as that is a rule I can follow. Having just a few Syns leads to me gorging uncontrollably.

Week Fifteen – The Big Picture

This week was the worst. Three and a half pounds gained. The word *'Gained'* is one of those jargon words like the other word I experienced in Week Six *'Maintained'*. Gained means that I am a complete failure and have no self-control. Gained means that I will never lose my weight. Gained means that my poor old heart will never experience a long and enjoyable life along with the rest of me. Gained is the pits.

Some definitions might be helpful here.

Maintained:
A dictionary definition for this is
'to keep in a specified state, position, etc.:'
My definition is *'To fail at losing more weight'*

Gained:
A dictionary definition for this is
'to acquire as an increase or addition:'
My definition is *'To fail utterly at life."*

Attain:
A dictionary definition for this is
'to reach, achieve, or accomplish; gain; obtain: to attain one's goals.'
My definition is the same as the dictionary's. I'm just not very good at this.

Miserable week. I can't even turn the pain into something positive. It has really knocked me back. Two helpful members who shall remain nameless (But their pseudonyms are June and Phillip) encourage me with the words *'Look at the big picture. You have done so well.'*
I admit in my better moments that this is in fact true. The big picture is that I have done very well with Slimming World. But that doesn't comfort me today.

Why have I gained this week? I refer you to the previous chapter on cheating. I am a Ninja cheater trained in the dark art of self-deception.

Week Sixteen –   The Plan

I now have my daily plan back in place. The depression of last week has lifted and I am set. I wasted Saturday and Sunday on being a morose, self-pitying slob. But I am good at Mondays. My favourite day of the week. I have planned my food for the next five days. I must thank Felicity who posted her week's menu in the Facebook group. Felicity is extremely focused and posts often in the Facebook group. Sometimes her happy attitude aggravates me, (My fault, not hers) but this time her food diary post was very helpful.

Monday

Breakfast: Overnight oats: A concoction of porridge oats, yoghurt and fruit left in the fridge overnight. It tastes better than it sounds and looks. (Full recipe Week Twenty-Five)
Lunch: Toast and Marmite, fresh apple.
Dinner: Spicy chicken curry on a bed of sweetheart cabbage (See Week Eighteen)
Snacks: Hi Fi Bar. Another piece of toast and Marmite. Slice of Scan Bran chocolate cake.

Tuesday

Breakfast: Overnight Oats: (Yes it does get boring)
Lunch: Cold meat with salad and yoghurt
Dinner: Spicy chicken curry remains from yesterday on a bed of rice and broccoli
Snacks: Slice of Scan Bran chocolate cake. Banana.

Wednesday

Breakfast: Overnight Oats: (Sorry!)
Lunch: Sandwiches, crudités and dips, sausage roll, two slices of cake – Buffet lunch at church - 20 Syns in all

Dinner: Leek and chicken risotto with sweetheart cabbage
Snacks: Slice of Scan Bran chocolate cake. Desperato beer at
snooker – 9 Syns

Thursday

Breakfast: Overnight Oats: (Really Sorry!)
Lunch: Bacon and cheese panini with side salad and diet coke
– pub lunch with wife & daughter – 24 Syns in all
Dinner: Fried egg on toast
Snacks: Slice of Scan Bran chocolate cake.
(This was a very bad 'speed' day)

Friday

Breakfast: Overnight Oats: (Must think of something different
for breakfast)
Lunch: Cold meat and salad. Apple and satsuma.
Dinner: Medallion beef steak with carrots, broccoli and
sweetheart cabbage.
Snacks: None – Getting weighed in the morning so trying not
to eat any more.

Even the two meals out were planned as I do these
regularly. i.e. buffet at church on Wednesday and pub lunch
on Thursday. I might as well factor them in. These five days
gave me a two-pound weight loss after the debacle of last
week. I'm back on track and feeling good about myself.

Week Seventeen – The Wisdom of Mandy-Lace

As the weeks have gone by I have come to realise that our glorious consultant, Mandy-Lace, is a lot sharper than she at first appears. She listens intently and you can see her brain working behind her eyes as she understands what is being said. This is particularly true with people's excuses. I can see her deciding whether to confront the excuses or to let them pass. I have witnessed this personally.

Behind her decision making is a strong, authentic desire to help us all in our struggle to lose weight. Sometimes it is better to come straight out and confront someone with the fact that their excuses are rubbish and even lies. Other times she lets it go and gives words of encouragement to the member. It is clear to me that she knows it all.

I usually think to myself that I want her to be brutally honest with me all the time, to help me speed up my weight loss. In fact, I am not always brave enough for the shout.

The wisdom of Mandy-Lace is that she knows. She truly knows.

Week Eighteen – Sweetheart Cabbage

There is a character in the Slimming World experience who has not been mentioned enough thus far. He sits on the central table at group every week. He is called the sweetheart cabbage. At Christmas, he even wore a Santa outfit.

I know I have just anthropomorphised a vegetable, but it is an important part of every meeting and now part of most days' menu for me and my nearest and dearest. You can eat almost as much as you like of this cabbage and no harm can come to you.

It can be eaten finely shredded and raw, or boiled in water lightly for a few minutes. Someone in our group has roasted it but I wouldn't do that. Roasting is for chicken, potatoes and parsnips, not cabbage. Sweetheart cabbage is a 'Speed' food which means that you should eat lots of it. Every meal should have at least a third of the plateful as speed food.

There are many other speed foods that I have learnt to love over the months. The main ones are carrots, celery, swede, broccoli, butternut squash, strawberries, mixed summer fruits, apples and satsumas.

The Day I Fell In Love With An Apple

Apples are displayed in packs of four or six in my local supermarket. They are sometimes put on special offer. But what they don't tell you is that they are not the best apples on sale. One day I was innocently looking for inspiration for snacks and I spotted a solitary box of Empire Apples sitting in the fruit section. You could pick them up and inspect them for blemishes and bruises. They were very large apples and bright, shiny red in colour. I proceeded to select the four best apples out of the box and placed them in a bag.

They were ridiculously expensive. About 65-75 pence each but I took the plunge and put them in the shopping trolley. When I got home I decided to eat one straight away.

The taste was extraordinary. Sweet and bitter and fresh and exhilarating. All at the same time. Forget chocolate treats and fried food, this is the best food in the world. I now keep a stock of Empire Apples for snacks. My second choice is Braeburn Apples. I urge you to splash out and buy the best apples out there.

The side benefit of this glorious new obsession of mine is that when I feel peckish and urgently in need of something to eat, I eat an apple, or even two.

Week Nineteen - Lost In Translation

This week I found myself looking for excuses. As my brain sought to say something intelligent to rescue my extreme disappointment at putting weight on, I uttered the phrase "I was expecting that." The only problem is, I wasn't expecting to stay the same weight. I was sure that I had been good and yet I had added half a pound on to my weight from the previous week.

As I uttered the phrase I acknowledged to myself the lie. I said it to cover my disappointment. There are in fact a number of well-worn phrases that I have noticed over the weeks that members use to disguise their true meaning. Here are some of them. They all follow a similar theme.

"I was expecting that." Means "I wasn't expecting that." This is a classic sorrowful phrase when you know full well that you have done your exercise and stuck to the plan but your body has decided to throw you a curve ball and not behave. I feel the pain of any member who comes to group genuinely thinking they have lost weight only to see the numbers on the dial prove otherwise.

"I'm not surprised." Means "I can't believe it!" This is very like the first excuse. For people who lose weight in chunks and then stay static for a few weeks. It can be heart-breaking.

"I'm happy with that." Means "I am totally disappointed with that." This harmless phrase usually ends up with some colourful language after two minutes as the increase in weight is inwardly digested and absorbed in the mind.

"I know I have put weight on this week." Means "I hope the scales are kind to me as I have cheated all week." You got yourself into this mess. Get yourself out of it. Not much sympathy.

"I had a feeling that something was wrong." Means "I am a complete Wombat and know exactly what I have been up to." Again, no tears of sympathy for this. Either you are on a diet or you are not. I'm too black and white in my thinking on this, according to my nearest and dearest.

"I have had a difficult week." Means "I decided from the first day of the week that there was no way I was going to follow the eating plan properly. I need a break." This excuse can be true and permissible if used in moderation. We all have tough times. But you cannot use it for more than five consecutive weeks and expect to be believed. Remember, Mandy-Lace knows everything.

"I'll take that." Means "After being so good this week I expected more, but the half a pound that the scales show is better than a maintain or a gain. I hate this diet but it's all I've got that works."

"I'm drawing a line under things." Means "I'm back to square one. Starting again from today."

"It's my star week". I bet it is. How many of those do you have in a month? (Not wishing to sound extremely unsympathetic as a mere male who still doesn't understand these things).

There are many more phrases that people use than this, but I haven't been able to translate them yet.

Week Twenty – Three Stones Award

Quite ridiculous. I'm not ready for this week yet. I lost a miraculous five pounds to achieve my three stones weight loss award. Smashed it in fact. Three stones, one and a half pounds. How did I do it? I wish I knew. The pain of the maintains and gains have worn me down to stop believing in the Slimming World diet. Now I am a true believer once more. How fickle I am. I am glowing with pleasure at the news, and I don't glow very much at my age.

Mandy-Lace asked me during the image therapy session to talk about what I have achieved. I gave the twenty second version of my story and received rapturous applause. I still cannot get used to the clapping.

I mentioned in week eight that I have a walking buddy, Rafe. Well unfortunately he has moved over to the dark side and got a bit obsessive with his walking. We have been doing between three and five miles each Tuesday evening. He has now enrolled himself in a charity walk along the River Thames from Oxford to Reading.

This walk is eighty-four kilometres long. That is two marathons' distance. This Tuesday he invited me to join him on the walk. I can't do this as my maximum is about 15 kilometres. But I did agree to sponsor him. He has been training heavily and going on a 36 kilometre and a 54 kilometre walk to get his distance up. I refrain from dampening his enthusiasm as I know his charity means a lot to him. But it is too far.

His charity is the brilliant Toilet Twinning organization. He is closely involved with this concern. He hoped to raise enough money to supply twenty-one toilets to places in the world that have no facilities. If you sponsor a toilet you get a photo certificate showing the toilet you have twinned with. These are all located in places of great need.

You can visit the charity at **toilettwinning.org**.

In the event, I dropped him off in Oxford and he completed the walk in a very fast time. But his feet were a mess afterwards as he hadn't factored in the possibility of rain. He had to wear Jesus sandals for a few weeks to recover. Not up to his usual debonair look. He successfully raised enough money for twenty-five new toilets. Flushed with success he is planning to do another sponsored walk in 2017.

He generously gave me a bottle of red wine for taking him to Oxford, which is about 30 syns in total. It was high alcohol content wine. He is not helping me, but I will struggle my way through it, glass by glass, and spread the syns out.

Week Twenty-One - The Bravest People Of All

This week someone came back to our Slimming World group having dropped out some months before. They had been a member when I started but had stopped coming to group. I remembered the lady because she has exactly the same name as a cousin of mine, Steph Maynard.

As she walked to the door I immediately welcomed her by name. She looked at me, surprised but grateful and congratulated me on my evident success with my weight loss. Steph always wears a massive shawl that she uses to hide her huge frame and her obesity. She had called Mandy-Lace in the week so she was expected. She had shame and blame written deep into her features.

I regret that a small corner of my brain condemned her as a fool for not staying to our group. Think how much lighter she would be if she had stayed to our group. Then I remembered that other people have their own monsters and dinosaurs to deal with in life. They are not the same as mine. Who am I to judge?

Some people come and go quite regularly. A sign of the inner struggles we all have, to keep to a diet. No one ever said it would be easy and this is the case for many occasional members.

As I mulled over Steph's reappearance I thought about her courage at first deciding to come back to group, and then going through with it. This morning she had made her decision to return and had got up extra early to walk over to Bluebrook Park Hall in good time. Then she had faced up to me, Mandy-Lace and the rest of the group. It must be so difficult to come back. I really admire people who return to group. They are the bravest people of all.

Week Twenty-Two –   Nothing Fits

I have no clothes that fit me anymore. My XXXL cheapy shirts from Direct Sports are like tents. My waist size 46" trousers from the supermarket are hanging off me and I have had to add new holes in my belt to stop them falling down. In my own private world, I am a fashion icon, and these oversized clothes are working against the image I am trying to portray.

I do have a stock of smaller sized trousers that my nearest and dearest has been storing up in a suitcase in the event that I might actually lose weight sometime. I am begrudgingly grateful to be reunited with them but I would rather have new stuff. The trouble with that is that it is a waste of money with so much more weight to lose. Baggy trousers for me for the foreseeable future.

In the first week Mandy-Lace told me to get a bit of string and use it as a measure around my waist. This bit of string is now showing a good five inches' spare length when wrapped around me. The problem is that I don't do pieces of string. I have resolved to buy a new smaller belt when the opportunity arises. I can then compare the belts rather than admire a bit of string.

One thing that is happening more and more now is that people are noticing my weight loss. I received some proper compliments about my success from someone I meet each week. One lady I know even told me I looked *'really good'*. I will not be telling Naomi about this.

Week Twenty-Three – Hi Fi Bars

The Slimming World people have a few food products of their own that they promote. One of these products is a range of Hi Fi Bars. These are tasty but a bit tiny for my appetite. One mouthful of flavour and they are gone. There are about six different flavours available at any one time. Phillip impressed us all one week by consuming a whole box of *'chocolate wonder'* at our group meeting before it had finished.

There is a bit of an issue however in that the people at head office keep introducing new flavoured ones and discontinuing the old favourites. Some members find that a favourite regular snack of theirs is taken away from sale never to be seen again. Each bar is worth about 3 syns each. Daniel, Mandy-Lace's other half sells them from a table by the entrance door.

His sales style must be acknowledged and recognised as laid back in the extreme. He sits quietly and unobtrusively by the table full of Hi Fi bars and awaits his customers patiently. And they come in their droves. He eagerly ticks off each sale against a sheet listing all the products. He easily sells sixty boxes each week. I'm thinking that there is good money in these Hi Fi bars. I have no idea if Mandy-Lace and Daniel profit from the sale of them but they do sell very well.

The product I buy almost weekly is the scan bran crispbreads. I use these to make a chocolate cake. This cake can be a lifesaver at about nine o'clock in the evening when we are getting peckish and needing a tasty snack. The scan bran is quite high in fibre, which helps to keep us regular, if you get my meaning.

Week Twenty-Four –   Big Business

It has not escaped my notice that Slimming World is big business. Even in our small corner of this world, Mandy-Lace has announced that we will be splitting our overlarge group into two groups to cope with the numbers of people attending. The groups will meet at eight thirty and ten thirty on a Saturday morning and we can choose which group we attend. I am going to go to the early meeting. I am a morning person. Naomi has no choice in the matter. Additionally, our area supervisor, Jacey, made a drop-in visit to ask for candidates to consider the career prospects for new Slimming World consultants.

There is not a rush of applicants to see Jacey following up this opportunity and I am not surprised. It is not a role suitable for everyone. But as a retired businessman I have started to see how the business works. This is not a bad thing, I'm just noticing it. For the right person, like Mandy-Lace, being a consultant would be a great opportunity to earn money while bringing up a family. I hardly pay attention to Jacey's presentation, safe in the knowledge that it is not for me.

Only last week I met a new consultant marketing her new group in the foyer of my local supermarket. She was giving out leaflets and chatting to people about the Slimming World plan. I introduced myself and told her I was in the Bluebrook Park group. She was really impressed with my weight loss so far and congratulated me. She also knew Mandy-Lace. I expect that all the local consultants have get togethers from time to time.

Then it occurs to me that my very own Naomi would be very good at it. Something to consider.

Week Twenty-Five – Payday

My twenty-four weeks of vouchers from Dr.Cody have run out this week and I have to pay for the first time. This is not irksome or very expensive. Being over sixty I get a special rate. But it does change my relationship with Slimming World.

Now I am no longer beholden to my wonderful GP who has sponsored me thus far. Now I am in it with both feet. I booked a twelve-week special deal that is available at the moment knowing that I hate wasting money by missing a week. It will keep me attending every week.

The Weekly Raffle

Each week there is a raffle. The proceeds from the raffle are used to provide the prize and pay for the free coffee and tea which is served in the group. Tom eagerly and very professionally sells the tickets at 10 pence for a ticket. I always buy 10 tickets, every week. Tom is the king of the raffle tickets selling. No one else does it as well. Especially not me.

And guess who won the raffle this week? Yours truly. The prize was a bag full of the ingredients to make 'Overnight Oats'. Added to this were a few other free vegetables and a sweetheart cabbage. I enjoy winning raffles and gratefully receive the bag full of goodies to take home.

Overnight Oats Recipe

It seems that everyone has their own method of making overnight oats. Let me share with you how I do it, which is of course the correct way.

Ingredients

40 grams porridge oats
1 pot of Muller light yoghurt – almost any flavour.
As many mixed fruit berries as you want. I use frozen mixed berries.

Method

First carefully weigh out the oats. Then thoroughly mix in the yoghurt. Then add the mixed fruit and combine it all together. Cover the mix and put it in the refrigerator. I usually use an airtight plastic container. The frozen fruit defrosts overnight and the recipe provides you with a great breakfast in the morning.

Week Twenty-Six – Social Team

Very early on in this journey (Second use of the 'J' word), my nearest and dearest decided that we would join the Social Team. This is a group of members who volunteer to help Mandy-Lace with the running and administration of the Bluebrook Park group. We signed up after about six weeks. Naomi was immediately asked to work on the 'Pay' computer where members pay their subs and sign in.

I was asked to be a Welcomer. Sometimes I replace Daniel selling the Hi Fi bars when he is away on business. I have also sold the raffle tickets that Tom usually sells. On the rare times he is absent I get his job. Only on one occasion did I get to attempt all three jobs in the same week. Welcoming, Hi Fi bar selling and Raffle tickets selling, all at the same time. It was a disaster and I never want to do that again. My head was spinning by the end of group.

There are secret benefits to being a Social Team member. I'm not sure if other people are supposed to know, but there are extras for helpers. On our 38th wedding anniversary Mandy-Lace came around with a huge bouquet of flowers to wish us well. She is so thoughtful.

We also receive books and magazines for free when there are spare ones. Then in August we had a huge Social Team barbeque at her home. A great night out. Apparently, we are being invited to a Slimming World do at Christmas as well. Another benefit is the friendship and camaraderie that exists within the Social Team members. We are becoming good friends.

Week Twenty-Seven – This Stuff Really Matters

I will not name anyone today; some things are too personal.

I am definitely not the person to help them, but I noticed two of the younger lady members arriving in tears today. I do not know them well and turned a blind eye as they composed themselves in the foyer. Not to put a gloss on it. Both these young girls have let themselves go and are extremely overweight. They should be happy go lucky, pretty young things enjoying life to the full and yet circumstances and bad decisions have thrown too much rubbish in their direction and they have to deal with it daily. This doesn't make my witness of their pain any easier. I try to think of a way I can help, and there is none.

I nodded towards Mandy-Lace and pointed out to her the two young ladies as they joined the queue. I could see from her expression that she knows them and their life very well. I am so relieved.

Over the weeks, I have discerned many of the secondary issues that people coming to group have to deal with. These are additional to being overweight. For some members, these issues are the prime cause of their problem with weight. Poor health, personal grief, relationship break-up, abusive relationships, mental health issues, post-traumatic stress and more.

Dealing with these life issues while trying to lose weight is nearly impossible, and yet many of the members are successful in doing so. The Slimming World diet is one area of life we can control even if everything else around us is going crazy. This stuff really matters. I have talked to some of the men who attend and spoken into some of their experiences but it is not really my place. With the ladies of the group I do not get involved with personal details.

Having said this I have ended up hearing some of the struggles, pain and grief of members' lives because they are so open about them. The very public location for this happening is the queue through the door while members are waiting to pay their subs and sign in. I am frequently humbled by peoples' honesty.

Week Twenty-Eight – Facebook Group

On reviewing the diary so far, I have noticed a huge omission. I have hardly mentioned that the Bluebrook Park Slimming World group has its own special group on Facebook. And you, dear reader, know nothing about it.

It is all a bit secret because you can only be on the Facebook group if you are a fully paid up member of the Slimming World group and Mandy-Lace allows you in. It appears to me that Mandy-Lace is a bit 'gung ho' with her permissions. She lets in everyone and even if they stop coming they are still there for a few months after they leave, reading about all our secrets.

Mercifully, not too many personal secrets are shared although sometimes there is too much earthy information for my liking. Some people post almost every day, others have weeks when they are alive on Facebook and then we don't see them for ages. It doesn't matter. The group offers support for members and it is a good point of contact. Mandy-Lace posts the results for the previous week recording all the awards and successes. She also posts motivational digital postcards to keep us on the straight and narrow.

The main thing posted by members is food. Photos of Breakfast, Lunch and Dinner. Along with these photos are recipes and cooking methods to help.

None of the food photos that other members post look as good as mine. Not even close. Am I the only one who thinks this?!...

Week Twenty-Nine – New People

Over the weeks there is a steady turnover of people who come through the doors. Some appear keen and eager for a week or two and disappear into the ether, never to be seen again. Others last a little longer. Then there are the determined members who stay with the plan and become a central part of the group. Let me tell you about some of them.

Tamsin has been there all the time. How could I forget? Tamsin oversees the pay station where members pay their subs and register their presence for the weigh in. Tamsin knows everything and with her head down works furiously for the first 40 minutes of the meeting to make sure the hordes of aspiring thin people are dealt with swiftly and efficiently. Her husband, **Alan**, also attends although I have to say he is as thin as a rake. He is there for Tamsin in the same way that Naomi is there for me.

Joan joined a few months after me and at first I didn't notice her. But then she started achieving good numbers with the scales and I took big notice. I always watch who is doing well because these people are cleverer than all the others. They do the diet and lose the weight.

Joan's husband, **Pierre**, has just joined up to support Joan. He doesn't need to lose very much weight. Both Joan and Pierre joined the social team from day one and Pierre took over the tea making duties from the excellent **Duke**, Mandy-Lace's father in law. Pierre's biggest achievement so far is to serve our coffee cold, having forgotten to boil the kettle.

Jemima brings her cute little daughter to group and is on a fast track to weight loss. She stays in the background but I have spotted her. She is focused and determined. Her friend, **Stan**, has also started coming. He is an obsessive Reading Football Club supporter. He knows everything there is to know about his team. He also rides everywhere on his bicycle including riding to group on a Saturday morning.

Felicity is also a keen Reading supporter attending the home games. Sometimes she attends our group in her Reading Shirt before rushing off to the game. Such dedication!

Week Thirty – 4 Stones Award

This is mad. Love it!

I have lost 4 stones.

Week Thirty-One – The World's Most Tattooed Lady

At the risk of openly revealing my own prejudices, I do not like tattoos. It must be an age or upbringing thing. I thought as a child that the only people who had tattoos were sailors and criminals. It has become obvious to me in the thirty weeks I have been coming to the Slimming World group that I am out of date. The problem is that I can't avoid staring at the tattoos. They jump out at me.

Today we had a visitor from another group. She must be the world's most tattooed lady. She walked into our group and from what I could see she had them everywhere. Neck, arms, shoulders, lower back (you could see these ones when she bent over), fingers, feet, legs and probably everywhere else. I didn't ask to see.

"Concentrate Jones!" I screamed to myself inwardly as I tried to give her the same even handed welcome as I give to everyone else. I think I got away with it. Then another younger lady walked in and said 'Wow' at the sight of the tattooed lady.

"I'm getting some done for myself this week. I can't wait". She told me with such gleeful enthusiasm that I retreated to the kitchen for a second, much stronger, cup of coffee. Being an observant chap over the last thirty weeks, I think that my nearest and dearest and I are probably the only group members who do not have a tattoo. What is the world coming to?

Week Thirty-Two – Holiday In Wales

We didn't go to group this week as we were on holiday. Self-catering in a Welsh cottage with our daughter and her boyfriend, my daughter's best friend and her little daughter, Evie. We have holidayed in Wales for many years. There is no mobile signal and almost no internet where we go. The connection is so slow that you might as well not bother with it. You are forced to live offline for a week and we love that aspect of it all.

We needed the break. Lots of lovely coastal walks and sea air. We revisited some of our favourite old haunts including the best beach in the world, Three Cliffs Bay. Even in the summer no one really goes there as there are no facilities and you have to walk for a long way to get to it. Naomi retrieved her Welsh accent within hours of arriving and went from sounding a bit Welsh to being unintelligible depending on what she was talking about.

The evenings were spent doing quizzes and playing games. I wonder where my daughter gets her voracious competitive character from? I can't imagine. We pretended to be grandparents to Evie which was loads of fun.

We were able to stay on our diet as we self-catered for most of the week. Shouldn't make a dent in our downward trend.

Week Thirty-Three – Body Magic

Mandy-Lace came up with a new quote today. I can't remember the exact words but it was something like...

'What you eat makes you look good on the inside, Exercise makes you look good naked'.

Quite shocking really. I am beyond looking good naked. That ship has sailed long ago. Nevertheless, there is a murmur of amusement and approval around the room.

I am now walking about thirty miles a week and four or five other members are also doing lots of regular exercise. We are all gold or platinum award winners for body magic. The exercise part of the Slimming World is the bit I understand the most.

But Mandy-Lace burst my exercise bubble today by saying that it is what we eat that matters the most. She told me that special studies prove this. Phillip, my back-row *'comrade at arms'* took my side in the discussion which I appreciated, but I sulked for the rest of the meeting. I do not like being wrong.

Later that night, and just to check, I looked in the full-length mirror. Hmmm...

Week Thirty-Four –   I Bring A Friend

I am still wallowing in the fact that I have lost four stones. To emphasise this, and to brag a little, I decided to take a bag of builder's sand weighing 56 pounds to group. The same amount as my weight loss to date. The only problem was, I couldn't lift it. I had to wheel it to group on a sack barrow. The irony of this was not lost to me or anyone else.

I announced that I had brought a friend with me and then wheeled out to view the sack of sand. Most members tried to lift the sack of sand and couldn't. But I had been carrying this excess weight around for years. No wonder my poor heart was complaining.

Week Thirty-Five – Mr Sleek Award

There are not many men in our group. This is a pity as we all need to lose weight and men can do it much faster than women. That is not to say that we don't have our own unique struggles. It is hard not to get unnecessarily competitive in any area of life. This does filter through to Slimming World but as there are so few of us it is not too hard to be the winner. In the main, Phillip and I win the battle of men's weight loss most weeks.

Today this is rewarded by the great honour of both of us becoming **Mr Sleek 2016**. We shared the award. The sophisticated side of me knows I should be crawling under a bus to hide, but I am not that sophisticated. I am totally chuffed. I think Phillip feels the same. We are awarded Slimming World branded desk top pens with a stand and smart red ties with "Mr Sleek" printed on them in black. We both decided to wear the red ties and fumbled over tying them properly. I can't recall the last time I wore a tie. We were both asked to share our weight loss story which we completed in a matter of moments. No point overdoing the speeches.

Mandy-Lace had photos taken which were later posted in the Facebook group. In my opinion I am still not slim enough for photos.

Clarice won the Ladies version of the award. Well deserved, although I voted for June. (Sorry Clarice). June came a very close second. Clarice's speech was just as short as mine and Phillip's. We moved on to the rest of Image Therapy.

I am looking for future opportunities to wear the Mr Sleek Tie. Do you have any ideas? I plan to wear it on Christmas Eve to our group but most people in the real world would do a double take at the sight of it and say 'Huh?'

Week Thirty-Six – I Mistakenly Post My Dinner

In the world of Facebook there are groups and there is your main timeline. It is important that you post the right stuff in the right place. Today I told all my 247 Facebook friends about my dinner tonight. I only meant to tell the people in the private Slimming World Facebook group.

This created a certain amount of confusion and unbridled mirth at my expense. The point is that I have told hardly anyone that I am on a diet. Only a few of my friends know about it because I see them most weeks and they have noticed my weight loss. My Facebook friends live all over the world, and due to the fact that I posted a photo and description of my dinner, they all now know about my diet.

They were not too unkind, but I like keeping things secret until I want the world to know.

Week Thirty-Seven – Well That Was Weird

I couldn't go to my own group this week as I had been invited to a Men's Breakfast on Saturday. I decided to visit another group to get weighed. I've always been a bit of an explorer and I love being nosey, so this was an easy opportunity to satisfy both these needs. There are many other Slimming World groups in Bracknell and yet again I see that this is big business. If all the groups are as large as ours then there must be 1,500 members for this diet system in Bracknell alone.

I found a group that meets on a Friday morning. It was about three miles walk from my house and I walked for my daily exercise session to get there. It was a bit weird. I felt some first morning nerves as I entered the room, but I didn't need to fear. One of the members spotted me and supplied me with a cup of coffee – strong, no sugar and only a dribble of milk.

The consultant, Eleanor, was very occupied with talking to people but still found time to have a twenty second chat with me. Everything in the group was the same but different. There was a pay station and a weigh station and Eleanor ran exactly the same format for the Image Therapy talk. But it wasn't quite the same feel as when Mandy-Lace does it. It was like saying the same words but in another language. I can't wait to go back to my group next week.

The Men's Breakfast on Saturday was a disappointing wash out as there was no fruit salad or anything else healthy on offer. I didn't want to risk the greasy spoon breakfast so I went hungry.

Week Thirty-Eight –   I Must Have Cheese

I miss cheese. You are allowed to eat cheese on the Slimming World diet but the portions are so small that they hardly touch the screaming appetite I have for cheese. Stilton, Danish Blue, Roquefort and any other blue cheese are my favourites. But in truth I could eat a barrel load of any type of cheese if I allowed it in the house. Because of this obsession with cheese I have avoided it completely for the whole year so far.

I must confess to a couple of other foodie obsessions. Peanuts, cashews, pistachios, walnuts, brazil nuts and more. As long as it looks like a nut I am nuts for them. The final evil I must avoid is cakes. I miss all the baking I used to do.

Other members talk longingly about chocolate but that specific obsession does not affect me at all.

Week Thirty-Nine – Food Optimising

Now is the time to relay to you what I eat daily. It has taken until now for me to fully grasp the eating plan. This is not a reflection on the diet being complicated. Rather it is me trying to relearn a lifetime of bad eating habits and advice.

Speed Food

The big thing for me is speed food. If my plate is full of fruit and vegetables of a certain kind that is a good thing. I have learnt to pile my plate high with sweetheart cabbage, carrots, swede, celery, salad leaves, cucumber, strawberries, raspberries, oranges, apples, melon, and so on. If I have these taking up most of my plate I don't have room for other things.

Free Food

Second in line are free foods. This includes other fruit and veg that are not speed food such as bananas and grapes. It also includes meat and eggs. I don't eat fish but this is free food as well. Then there is rice, pasta, quinoa, couscous, potatoes and the like. You can eat unlimited amounts of free food but of course if your plate is full of speed food there isn't much room left on the plate.

Healthy 'A' food

This was the part that totally confused me in the early days. These are measured portions of things like milk, cheese, yoghurt and other things. You are allowed one healthy 'A' per day.

Healthy 'B' food

This includes bread, cereals and crispbreads. You are allowed one of these healthy 'B' foods per day.

Syns

Everything else is syns and you must count them accurately in your day. Mandy-Lace informs you in your first week what your syn allowance is per day. My allowance is twenty-five syns per day. I hardly ever get close to this number. Any food or drink can be called syns. Chocolate, alcohol, cheese – literally anything. But you have to measure correctly and be honest with the portion sizes.

We are supposed to savour and enjoy our syns. I always feel like the bad boy in class when I indulge in them.

The big thing that I do differently now than when I started is the portion sizes. I go wild with the quantities of speed food but have reduced my portion sizes on everything else. That works for me.

I sometimes get hungry but this usually means that I have forgotten a meal or haven't had time to cook.

Our Food Choices

To see how this translates into meals, here are our main choices for Breakfast, Lunch and Dinner. Naomi and I are very much creatures of habit and tend to stick to the same sort of meals each week. Occasionally we have a rush of blood to the head and cook something different, but at our age this is very rare indeed.

I try to make sure that all food is prepared from scratch but as you will see we sometimes have to use ready pre-packed stuff if we have no time to cook.

All our bread is homemade from 100% Wholemeal Stoneground flour.

Breakfast Choices
- Porridge with a dollop of jam or golden syrup ('Dollop' is one of my favourite words of the English language. Dollop!)
- Overnight oats
- Bacon Sandwich with a fried egg on top. (This is our version of a recipe from the 'Spanglish' Movie – Great movie by the way).
- Full English breakfast including sausages, bacon, egg, baked beans and toast.
- Selection of fresh fruit.

Lunch Choices – The hardest meal of the day to sort out.

- Mugshot and fresh fruit
- Chickpea Dahl Loaf with salad– A glorious Slimming World recipe
- Cold Meat and Mixed salad
- Mixed fruit salad
- Ready meal from the Healthy Extras range at Tesco or the Slimming World range from Iceland
- Toast and Marmite with fresh fruit.

Dinner Choices – Our favourite recipes

- Chilli Con Carne on Sweetheart cabbage
- Chicken/Lamb/Beef Curry on rice and speed food. (Lots of different types of curry choices)
- Chicken and leek risotto with broccoli
- Medallion Beef Steak with Slimming World chips and speed food.

- Homemade multi-vegetable soup with homemade wholemeal bread rolls.
- Shepherd's pie using swede/parsnip/squash for the mash.

Snacks and Syns (A mix of the following items if needed to supplement our main meals)

- Glass of wine – most days
- Scan Bran chocolate cake – Slimming World recipe
- Fig and Pistachio Biscotti biscuit
- Apple
- Banana
- Dry toast with jam or marmite
- Hartley's low sugar jelly with mixed fruit and low fat spray cream
- Muller light yoghurt – almost any flavour

Regular Cheats and Naughty Days – (I'm being transparently honest here)

- Another glass of wine
- Occasional beer when I play snooker
- Piece of cake on a Wednesday evening at our church housegroup
- We sometimes eat out. I mostly order the best possible but sometimes it has to be burger and chips. I can't help myself. Naomi is always well behaved when we eat out. She must be an angel.
- Wednesday buffet lunch – could be almost anything and I can't resist free food.
- Thursday lunch out with my wife and daughter – I usually allow 24 Syns.

Week Forty – Flying Off The Shelf

The time has come for me to own some new clothes. I am generally a reluctant shopper but must agree that my baggy look can no longer continue. Naomi took me to my favourite tailor, which masquerades as a general supermarket every other day of the week.

I started at waist size 46 inches forty weeks ago. Now my size 40-inch waist trousers feel too big. We go to the menswear aisle to find waist size 38 inches. There are hundreds of pairs of trousers that could potentially fit me. I have choice, which I am not used to. I selected two pairs of jeans and a smart pair of trousers and retired to the changing room. It probably took me ninety seconds of careful thought and deliberation to pick them out from the rack.

They all fitted me perfectly. There was no extra tension from me breathing in while I did the belt up. My one inch *'balcony'* was quite tolerable in them although it still needs some work. (**The Balcony** is a technical term for the amount of belly overhang you have above your belt). We bought them all. The best pair were the *'Slimfit'* black jeans. I can't stop wearing them. I need to wear them all the time. Did I mention that they are *'Slimfit'*? Naomi must ask my permission before she washes them as I then have to wear something else.

Week Forty-One – Crash Test Dummies

Following a diet is extremely difficult. If it was easy, then the multimillion pound slimming industry would not exist. This week I watched one of our members metaphorically crash headlong into a wall. I heard them say that they were giving up as there was no point them attending each week, paying their fees and then not following the diet.

For this lady, life has got in the way of her good intentions. I do not know what has happened in her life but it has driven her to despair and made her give up trying to lose weight. I cannot blame her for it. I have been there myself.

You eat and eat and eat even though you know it is wrong. I hope more than I expect the lady to have second thoughts and comes back next week. I have witnessed this crashing process a number of times over the months I have attended my group. It is not pleasant to watch.

The App and Team Competition

Everything has an app these days. Even Slimming World. During the image therapy session people look up syn values in the app on their mobile phones. The first to speak out the syn value wins points for their team.

The teams are decided on an ad hoc basis, left half of the room and right half of the room. There are points awarded for people who gain awards. There are also points arbitrarily awarded by Mandy-Lace for recipes and contributions of value. At the end of the meeting the scorer for the winning team wins a prize.

If none of this makes sense you must come to the Bluebrook Park group one day to observe it all. The team competition can become highly animated at times.

There is a serious side to the app which is useful when you are away from home or out for a meal and you need to look something up. It will also record your progress on a weekly basis.

There is also a main website with thousands of recipes which you can use. This website showcases people who have completed their weight loss. These are very inspirational and I frequently find myself reading the life stories to gain encouragement for myself.

Week Forty-Two – Taster Days

Every now and then Mandy-Lace plans a taster day where we are encouraged to bring in food we have prepared that fits in well with the Slimming World diet. This is a very good way of trying out new things. You also learn of recipes and ideas that you would never have thought of.

I always try and bake something from one of the recipes on the Slimming World website. This week I cooked a Fig and Pistachio Biscotti recipe from the new Christmas recipe book. This turned out to be one of the best recipes I have tried out so far.

Delia baked some fantastic Eatabix cake and Laurie completely killed it with her Lemon Drizzle cake. I like sweet things in the morning and struggled with the many excellent savoury things on offer. But I did try Nigella's Houmous and Phillip's Chicken Curry. It is amazing what you can eat with Slimming World.

Week Forty-Three – Drugs and Pills

My latest health review brought with it a few surprises and some good news. I am slowly getting better. There is no promise of full recovery but getting better is good. One of my really bad pills had been halved in dosage by Dr. Cody some months ago. Today I was negotiating whether I could drop it completely along with another horrible drug.

I know I needed these drugs straight after my operation but I wanted to come off them if it was at all possible. I am now struggling with the side effects which make me giddy and light headed. These symptoms have forced me to stop my daily walking while I sort out the problem.

In the following weeks, I had two sessions of tests with the nurses in my surgery, then I met up with Dr. Cody for his reply to my request.

Just a year ago, my surgeon, Dr. Paul, had placed a note on my file to review my medication after twelve months. We are all singing from the same hymn sheet here. Dr. Cody agreed to let me come off the two drugs and to have follow up tests a few weeks later to check everything out.

The NHS is getting terrible press coverage at the moment, but I can only praise it. The care and service I have received over this year has been exemplary.

As soon as I am off the drugs for a week I am much recovered and start my walking again. I might not die just yet. I hope I live.

Week Forty-Four – Ground To A Halt

I can no longer lose weight. No matter what I do, I go up and down like a yoyo. Mandy-Lace calls it the wiggly route to weight loss. I call it rubbish. Why am I saying this? Because since week thirty I have not managed to lose my next stone. It is worse than that. I haven't managed the next half stone. Up a pound, down a pound, round and round I go getting nowhere. With Christmas looming and no chance of being good over the festive period I think my next weight loss will have to wait for the new year. Very frustrating.

Martina seems to have a secret document that tells you a way of kick-starting your body back into losing weight. Mandy-Lace has let her borrow it for two weeks. This innocent looking 'dossier' obviously holds secrets that only a few members are allowed to see. I peer over Martina's shoulder but can't quite read what is on the pages. Her mum, Nigella, is also a bit quiet and shady about it, which makes me even more suspicious.

There is a hidden world within a world going on here and I want to know all its secrets. NOW!

Week Forty-Five – 365 Days

Today's group meeting coincided with the exact anniversary of my heart operation last year, 365 days ago. I attended the group meeting on my own as for the third week running. Naomi has the worst cough virus in history. She is bed ridden.

I can't stop thinking about this important anniversary today. It is a big day for me. I can still see in my mind all the doctors and nurses around the operating table if I close my eyes and think about it. Two anaesthetists, three nurses, two other people who I am not sure what their job was. Then there was a specialist surgeon brought up from Portsmouth in case my keyhole surgery didn't work and I needed emergency open heart surgery. She had her own team of two other people waiting on the side. I recall Dr. Paul telling me that I could watch what was happening on the monitor as they drilled out and repaired my blocked artery. Being awake for my operation was bad enough, I couldn't watch it on the tele.

I could feel the drilling inside me as it took place. The medical staff were inordinately happy in their work. The emergency second team on standby were not needed and they left after about forty-five minutes. Dr. Paul told them to go. I stayed put while he completed the operation. I think the whole thing was over in about ninety minutes.

I was taken to a ward and told to lie still for eight hours on my bed with no pillow. Eight whole hours lying still and flat with NO PILLOW! Agony. The nurses kept coming in every hour to check my wounds *'down there'*. That was a day I will never forget.

In our group today, Mandy-Lace handed pieces of paper out and asked us to write down something we were proud of. I wrote that I was proud of my weight loss since my operation and proud of the improvement in my health generally. We then screwed up these bits of paper into 'snowballs' and threw them onto the central table.

One by one the messages were read out. There were many extremely touching and deeply moving statements read out that morning. When it came to mine most people guessed who had written it. I quietly announced that it was exactly a year since my op. I swallowed a massive lump in my throat with a determined gulp. No tears, but for a split second it was dangerously close.

Week Forty-Six – An Epic Day

This truly was an epic day. Christmas Eve 2016. And the room was almost full of people trying to breath in and look like they have been good in the run up to Christmas. Not only that, some people had lost weight, myself included. One and a half pounds. Considering my recent heavy social calendar that is a miracle.

The last two weeks of my life has been a blur of festive food. Mince pies, sausage rolls, fruit cake, turkey dinners, double cream and much more.

Mandy-Lace invited me during the week to bring my guitar so that we could sing some Christmas songs in the meeting. It went quite well even though not everyone sang. I have noted these miserable people's names down for future reference.

Most people did however get into the Christmas spirit of it all and it was a great morning. We played a party game and Mandy-Lace didn't do the Image Therapy session in the same way. Everyone promised that they were going to be good over the Christmas holidays, myself included.

It was never going to happen!

Week Forty-Seven – An Epic Day For All The Wrong Reasons

I told you it was never going to happen!

News Year's Eve group meeting and all those who are sober have turned up to be weighed after a week of overeating. The best laid plans we all promised were thrown out of the window, as we all ate and drank ourselves into oblivion over the festive period. I walked 20 miles this week but that hardly made a dent in my weight. I gained five and a half pounds. And there were others in the room who had put on more than that.

Martina, Nigella and I worked out that the group has cumulatively put on almost a whole person in weight gain this week. One hundred and nine pounds. Something to be proud of – not.

Three traitors to the cause actually lost weight. This included my nearest and dearest and the ever-faithful June. I can't remember who the other person was, I was so stunned.

Week Forty-Eight – First Meeting of 2017

I had already thought to myself in the week that there could be some new people coming today. I was thinking new year's resolutions and things. It turned out to be true. There were fifteen new people today who had signed up. As well as this, another ten prodigals from 2016 had returned to face the scales and re-start their diet. It was a packed-out room full of good intentions. There was a similar turn out for the second group. Mandy-Lace has got her work cut out in January keeping up with us all.

Instead of running a new members' group this week Mandy-Lace ran through the basics of the Slimming World diet with all of us. It was amazing how much I didn't know. Still it was good to hear the whole eating system laid out clearly step by step. There were lots of good questions and answers during the hour. Next week we will be back to our normal schedule.

The secret *'dossier'* that Martina had hidden away before Christmas is now in my hands and I am not letting go of it until Mandy-Lace reveals its secrets. It transpires that it is a special version of the diet that has been produced for people who have got stuck at a certain weight. Well that is me hands down. I have been dithering for fifteen weeks on this diet and getting nowhere.

There are sparse instructions which means that there are few things you are allowed on this version of the diet. But it is *'Guaranteed'* to kick start your body into action and restart the weight loss process.

As I read through the secret dossier I can see that committing to it will be extremely tough. But I am determined to complete what I have started and lose all my excess weight. I asked Mandy-Lace how many points I can consume. The answer is 25.

For you as my reader this is meaningless, but for me this means a bit more food through my mouth and into my tummy each day than I had expected. Halfway through the week Mandy-Lace 'WhatsApped' me (Don't you love apps and the verbs they create!) to say that I am permitted 31 points a day. She got the number wrong in the first place.

I resubmitted my diet plan to take account of this. The most important addition to my daily intake of food was a glass of wine which is 2 points for 125ml. I quickly consider the merits of drinking a whole bottle of wine per day and then calculating the remaining points that I can eat. A full bottle of wine would be 12 points. This would leave 19 points for food each day. Not bad. I am, however, still thinking like a fat person. I am not cured of my obsession with overeating yet.

The idea of this fast track version is to do it for a maximum of two weeks and then return to standard food optimising. By Wednesday I am fighting the urge to cheat. It is very hard to limit my food so strictly. Looking at my diet sheet plan it looks like a lot of food. But this is misleading. The portions are very small and there are hardly any carbs in the diet.

I resolved to force myself to behave for seven days and then review it. If I lose a good amount of weight on Saturday, then that will be all the encouragement I need to do a second week.

Week Forty-Nine – Anticipation

I have been six days on the fast track version of the diet. I also walked my regular Friday walk from Bagshot to Bracknell. Eight miles with a drop in to a friend's house halfway for a cup of coffee. I know I haven't wavered from the diet plan one iota. No cheating, no second guessing, nothing. I am expecting a good loss in the morning.

I want it to be the morning now so that I can get it over and done with. The next sentence will tell you the result, but please bear in mind that I have had to wait sixteen very nervous and tense hours before writing them…

…A bit of a letdown, three and a half pounds lost this week. I was hoping for five or six. My plan for the whole year was to get to five stones weight loss in total. Now, I have lost four stones five and a half pounds. I have eight and a half pounds to go in three weeks.

This is a very tough target. Basically, three pounds each week for the next three weeks. I have never done that yet.

Week Fifty – A Battle For The Mind

Definitely a *'good news, bad news'* week. I achieved my four and a half stones award. But I only just made it. With two weeks to go to my full year on the diet I am assured that I will not quite hit the five stones milestone. But I will be very close. I have seven more pounds to lose to achieve my goal.

I have two major battles to overcome. One with my body and one with my mind. I am not one of those people who can lose weight easily. I fight to lose weight and it can be very difficult when my body does not respond. Every now and then I read about someone who joined Slimming World and lost six stones in six months. That is not me! I am not like that person. Not even close. I have to fight for every pound of weight loss.

There was a definite sense of determination with most people in the room today. The Christmas festivities are well and truly gone and forgotten. Lots of promises were made and plenty of resolve expressed. But losing weight is not that simple.

Sophie had fire in her eyes as she told me she had put on half a pound. She was so furiously livid that she didn't stay to the group meeting. She was not sure that she wouldn't lash out verbally to us all and to Mandy-Lace. I fully understand her predicament. Her head dropped as she forthrightly and pointedly aimed for the door and rushed off.

I am sure that Sophie suffers the same battle for the mind that I do. The only difference for me now is that I have more confidence in this diet process. I know it works. But it doesn't work as well as I would like. It also doesn't work in a straight line. That is what creates the mind games in my head.

I think I can outwit my body by eating properly and doing lots of walking, but my body has a mind of its own and will only lose weight when it is good and ready. My body has its own schedule but it doesn't inform me about it. There is a huge disconnect here. Why does my body not behave?

Then I remember the pain and toil I have put my body through over the last 35 years and realise that I am part of the problem. Skinny thin people will have no idea what I am referring to here.

I am obsessed with food! I think about it all the time!

Once breakfast is over I am already thinking about what I am going to eat for lunch. After lunch I am fretting about my dinner. The only way to reduce my concern and worry about food is to plan carefully. This puts my obsession to rest till the next day because I have the comfort in my brain that more food is on its way. I don't think that I will ever be able to maintain my weight without careful planning. Then I must stick to my plan.

I do not understand skinny thin people who eat anything they like on a whim and a fancy. They never put on weight. Maddening!

There is a situation that occurs most weeks in my life and that is free food. Not free in the diet sense, but food I haven't paid for. If I am offered food that I haven't paid for, I feel obliged to partake. This happens every Wednesday when I attend a buffet dinner at church. (I must be there because I run the meeting). But there are other opportunities for free food most weeks. Men's meetings, neighbours' invites and many other regular occasions. I can barely stop myself from tucking in and gorging on all the free food available.

The World of Slimming

There will be some deep psychological reason for all this but I can't afford the therapy sessions to find out what it all means. Even if I went, I know I would never be cured.

Footnote: This diary entry was typed into my computer in about 4 minutes, a mad frenzy of keyboard activity. I do not think I will edit it as it gives an insight into the craziness in my head I feel when I am trying to lose weight and stick to a diet. I am not exaggerating when I call it a battle for the mind.

Please continue to next week's entry. It will be much better edited than this one.

92

Week Fifty-One –   My New FattBitt

I have a new watch. But it is so much more than a watch. It is like Big Brother, think George Orwell and his classic book, '1984'. I studied this book as part of my A level English in 1973. I never expected to be living it.

All my FattBitt friends can see when I am walking and when I am not. I can also keep an eye on them. This sort of openness is not easy to assimilate. I am not sure I want them all to know.

My friends are all ladies in the Slimming World group. Come on guys. I need some male competition and banter here. There was a five-day challenge that Felicity set up. At one point I was in the lead but two people have overtaken me. Here is the leaderboard as of 25th January 2017, at 23.07.

Kath	53,789 steps
Fern	53,264 steps
Ken	45,276 steps
Lane	43,477 steps
Felicity	42,787 steps
Jackie	33,601 steps
Rose	27,164 steps
Clare	24,192 steps
Celine	19,044 steps
Davina	15,863 steps

Even as I have typed this I spotted Rose surreptitiously putting in some late-night steps. Naughty, naughty Rose. It must be past your bedtime. I plan to go on a long walk tomorrow to restore my lead.

Stop Press: I did top the leaderboard for a while on Thursday, but Fern looks determined not to be beaten. Kath also appears to be a threat to my Challenge domination.

Week Fifty-Two – My Six Top Tips For Success

I am frequently asked by people how I have lost the weight and what is the best way to do the Slimming World diet. So here are my six top tips.

Stick to the plan 7 days a week

You can stick to the plan or not. But why would you waste money and effort on something you do not follow through on. Only serial dieters like myself know the reasons. I refer you back to the chapter on cheating. I am much better at sticking to the plan now. The two weeks of fast track helped me refocus and set myself up for the second year.

Major on speed food

You can be obsessed with speed food and this is a good thing. Just make sure you mix and match what you eat. There is no point turning your body into a wind farm and only eating cabbage and brussels sprouts. Look at all the speed foods that are permissible and then buy them. Then eat them. Don't wait for the sell by date to expire.

Speed food should be eaten fresh. I choose my speed food first when I plan a meal. I admit that this has only been true for the last few months or so. I am finally 'getting' the prime importance of speed foods.

Stay to group

I stay to group every week. Why wouldn't I? I've paid for it. In the three weeks I missed due to holidays etc., I felt as though I was missing a limb. I was desperate to get back to the group the following week. The people who stay to group lose the most weight. The people who do not stay to group lose less weight. It is a simple fact.

Nevertheless, there are people who do not stay to group, ever. Of course, there will be weeks when there is something more pressing that needs attending, but I plan my weekend around my Slimming World group time. I wouldn't have it any other way.

Don't beat yourself up

Things go wrong. If losing weight was easy we wouldn't be here. I no longer punish and berate myself when I fail. I acknowledge the fact and get back on the task of following the plan.

Set goals with dates

My first target was to lose 7 stones. I had no idea how long this would take. Well I now know that it will be more than a year. Because of this, I reset my target to lose 5 stones in the first year. The date for me to do this by is February 4th 2017. You will find out in the next chapter if I made it. If I do hit my target, fantastic. If I fail, then I still have the comfort that the goal helped me towards my long-term target.

Having a dated, achievable goal has helped me stick to the diet.

Be a positive person

I have a positive attitude. I made a decision years ago to see the best in people. Anyone can do this, it just takes practice and determination. Most positive emotions can be fueled by a decision to do the right things, make the right decisions and have the right attitude. Do it in cold blood and eventually the true character and feelings will be part of you automatically.

Review - Couple of the Year

Well that was disappointing. Half a pound loss in a week where I had stuck to the plan and done lots of body magic. For the whole year my weight loss was four stones eight and a half pounds. Not the five stones I set as my goal.

I know I will get there. But I am not there yet. I have decided to not cheat this weekend but stay on the diet which is actually a big step. It is so easy to make excuses to use Saturday and Sunday as a buffer before returning to the diet on Monday. I am beginning to win some of the mind games in my head.

Today was a major taster day and the food on offer was fantastic. Highlights were Laurie's Ginger Cake, Nora's Chocolate mousse, Delia's Chickpea Dahl Loaf, Candice's Egg and Ham muffin, Sophie's rather posh Ombré Raspberry Slice, Fern's Key Lime Pie, Mandy-Lace's Diet Cola Chicken with rice and much more. There was so much to eat that I cancelled breakfast and just stuffed on the free food on offer.

This was also the one year anniversary of me starting on my Slimming World journey. (Last use of the 'J' word). Looking back, I know I have done well. I have hopefully added years to my life and am well enough to enjoy it more.

Added to all this Naomi and myself were awarded couple of the year. There were about six couples nominated but we had the most votes. This was very humbling for us to know that our weight loss was recognised by others in the group. I gave a short speech and Naomi spoke about my brush with death with my heart. It was a bit emotional and moving for us all I think.

The Future

How do I see things for the next year?

Well firstly I have confidence that I will hit my target of seven stones weight loss this year. I know it will happen. Secondly, I do not ever see us stopping this diet. We will continue doing it for life.

I am going to keep writing my diary each week chronicling my weight loss story. This book of the first year will be published in about a months' time. I see it as a thank you gift to the members of Bluebrook Park Slimming World group.

They still don't truly realise how their lives and ours have worked together for my success. I'll keep telling them and maybe they will fully understand one day. We truly appreciated being voted 'Couple of the Year'.

We have some major changes in our circumstances happening this year which I will not talk about now. Suffice to say that the adventure of our life together continues apace.

If you have been touched or moved by this diary, please contact me. I would love to hear from you.

You can contact me through this website:

TheWorldOfSlimming.com

Other books written by Ken Jones

Guilty Until Proven Innocent

An 80's British rock star accused of multiple counts of sexual assault? Oh yeah, he's got to be guilty...right?

When former bad boy rocker turned reformed Christian businessman, Tom Harwell, is suddenly accused of sexual assault, he is stunned beyond belief. After up-and-coming news reporter, Lindi Loukas, starts a campaign to smear his reputation, his name is immediately dragged through the mud by the court of public opinion. Sure, Tom made mistakes in his past but not this one. This is all nothing but a big misunderstanding, it's got to be. He is a different man today - a better man, even - but when it comes to the media and newspapers, you can never seem to get away from your past...

But as Tom works to clear his name, everything starts to spin wildly out of control. With Ms. Loukas on the warpath to make a name for herself by any means necessary, anyone who threatens the fast-track of her career is in danger - but most especially Tom Harwell's name is on the top of her list.

Can Tom stop Lindi from completely trashing his name? Or will he forever be guilty with no chance to prove he's innocent?

The book has no foul language and no explicit details. It is a "clean" read and the first book in the "Lindi Loukas Reports" series.

The Memoirs of Edward Rochester

The Memoirs of Edward Rochester is a delightful re-telling of the amazing novel *Jane Eyre* by Charlotte Bronte. Re-imagined from the perspective of Edward Rochester, for the first time readers can learn his point of view and motivations. This book exposes Mr. Rochester's innermost thoughts, such as: how does an obnoxious tyrant fall in love? Why did Jane have such an effect on him? How did he come to grips with his past and open his mind enough to allow Jane to capture his heart? And the list goes on and on...

All of these questions and so many more are answered within newly created scenes - as well as alternate interpretations of the original ones - all finely crafted to invite new insight and exploration into this classic tale.

Books by Naomi Davies

'Sandy Wrighton and Friends' – A series of short romantic novels

Book One - Healing Love

Clair's whole life has been governed and controlled by a strict religious upbringing. Her parents now have a plan for her life, but this plan does not take account of her prodigious talent for singing.

Max is wild and free. He is alive and out of control. Max lives for the moment and lets nothing hold him back.

The lives of these two completely different young people collide with unexpected consequences and eventually with tragedy. Can love heal the pain of broken memories?

Book Two - A Maldives Adventure

After a roller coaster year, Sandy and Anne decide that they need a holiday. Nothing quite goes to plan however, and things start to go wrong even before they have boarded their flight. Nevertheless they do eventually arrive safely and discover an island full of secrets and mysterious people.

Most strange of all are the two perfect men, Paulo and Giorgio, who look like they are on holiday but keep disappearing with little or no explanation.

No one in this book is quite who they seem. Will Sandy and Anne find romance on the Emperor Island Hotel? Why is everyone so secretive and behaving so strangely?

Book Three - For The Love Of Music

Anne Richardson was beautiful and alluring. She didn't even have to work at it. She always looked good. This tended to stop all but the bravest of men approaching her. Ed was that bravest of men. But he was brash, unshaven, unkempt and with straggly uncut hair. More than that, he had been severely injured in Afghanistan and was now recovering from multiple wounds and a missing right leg. There is no way that these two people could fall in love, was there?

Book Four - The Welsh Victorian Dolls Mystery

Fiona Makin loved her little antique shop. It was in a sleepy English village and it was her whole life. She was far too involved with her business to fall in love! That was until she was dramatically rescued from being run over by a car.

Her saviour was the mysterious William Ayres. He was enigmatic, evasive and full of secrets. Could these two busy people stop working so hard and find time to fall in love?

Book Five - The Absent Bridegroom

After a troublesome holiday romance and an extremely difficult engagement Sandy is ready to be married to her love, the magnificent Paulo. The church was booked and the guests invited. The only trouble was that with ten days to go to her special day, he has disappeared. Will Sandy find him in time?

Colourblindness – The Unwritten Code – *A Parent's Guide to Colourblindness.*

Naomi Davies is an author from the UK who is Colour Blind. As she tells her family story, which has three generations of people who are Colour Blind, you will learn how to help your child if they are also Colour Blind.

This book takes the mystery out of Colour Blindness. It Explains how Colour Blindness affects people in their daily lives. You will also find how Colour Blindness is Inherited.

Printed in Great Britain
by Amazon

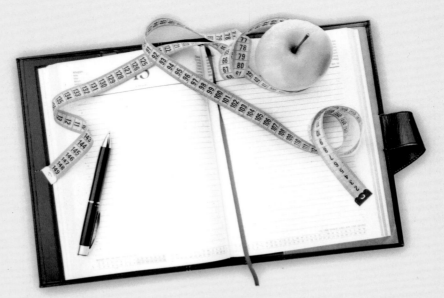

You know those celebrity weight loss books that make it seem like all you have to do is work out with your personal trainer, eat your perfectly portioned, personal chef prepared foods, be perfectly disciplined and the weight just magically falls off? Well, no, this is not that kind of book. Nope. What you have here is a book for the non-celeb, the everyday person with everyday weight loss issues.

The person who struggles with their weight and might have problems committing to a new and healthy lifestyle.

The person who needs to make a change but just needs a little push.

The real person who just needs a little encouragement from another real person who took charge of their weight loss journey and found real-life success.

This is that kind of book.

Follow along as the author gives you a candid look into the diary of his weight loss journey. Within the pages, read his private thoughts, musings, anecdotes and frustrations about what it's really like to struggle with finding the right balance of creating a healthier lifestyle and making those changes work. Real life, real problems, real hunger. He's right there with you.

Feel free to laugh, cry and even get frustrated as you read but by the end, you will be encouraged. Are you ready to be inspired to make those healthier lifestyle changes in your life? If so, this book can help you get there...

ISBN 9781543186574

9000

9 781543 186574

beginner's guide to rearing

Wild Birds

Third Edition

Samantha Bedford